Y0-CPB-542

Published by:
Lessons for Children, LLC
P.O. Box 632
Hinsdale, IL 60522
www.lessonsforchildren.com

Copyediting by Rosanne Cornbrooks Catalano

Special thanks to Gina DeConti of Imaginative Studios
www.imaginativestudios.com

Special thanks to Michael LaDuca of Luminus Media
for assisting in all aspects of this project.

ISBN: 978-0-9827739-0-1

LCCN: 2010907613

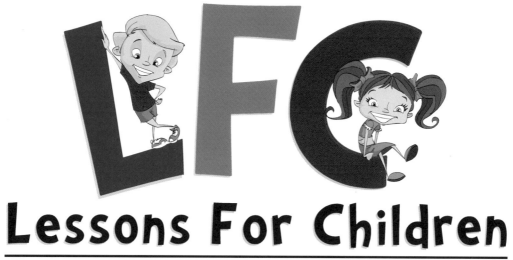

Lessons For Children

"It's up to us"

Written by: Antonio Braccioforte

Illustrated by: Matthew M. Keown

DEFINITION

mod•era•tion (mäd'ər ā'ѕhən)

1: avoidance of excesses or extremes

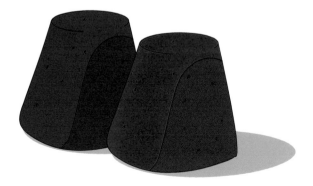

FROM ONE PARENT TO ANOTHER

In developed countries across the globe, the prevalence of childhood obesity has more than doubled or tripled, depending on the age group, within the past decade.

Health and nutrition begin at home. In order to teach your child moderation, it is important to set the right example. Children are very visual and absorb most of their knowledge through their eyes and ears. Also, children show more enthusiasm for their meals when they can be actively involved in their food choices.

Education is essential in this phase of their lives. To teach your children about fruits and vegetables, try to get them involved. You can do that by growing a garden, taking them to the grocery store, or choosing a recipe from a cookbook.

Avoid banning treats; remember, growing children need snacks to eat between meals. Rather, create your own, healthier snacks. The Internet is a great resource for researching healthy homemade treats for your child.

Keep in mind that eating in moderation can not only prevent obesity in children, it can also lower the risk of developing heart disease or diabetes as they grow older.

I am truly passionate about health and nutrition. I hope you enjoy reading this book as much as I enjoyed writing it.

Sincerely,

Antonio Braccioforte
"It's up to us!"

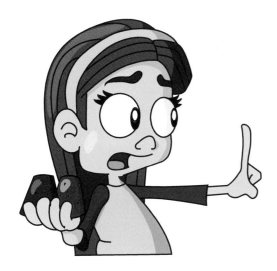
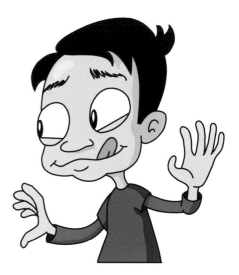

Before you begin reading 'In Moderation' ask your child…

- What is his or her favorite food
- Why they enjoy it so much
- How does it make them feel
- Explain the importance of a well-balanced meal
- Ask if they can define 'moderation'
    - o   If so, ask them to explain it to you
    - o   If not, explain 'moderation'

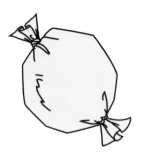
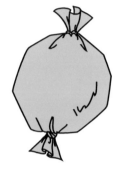
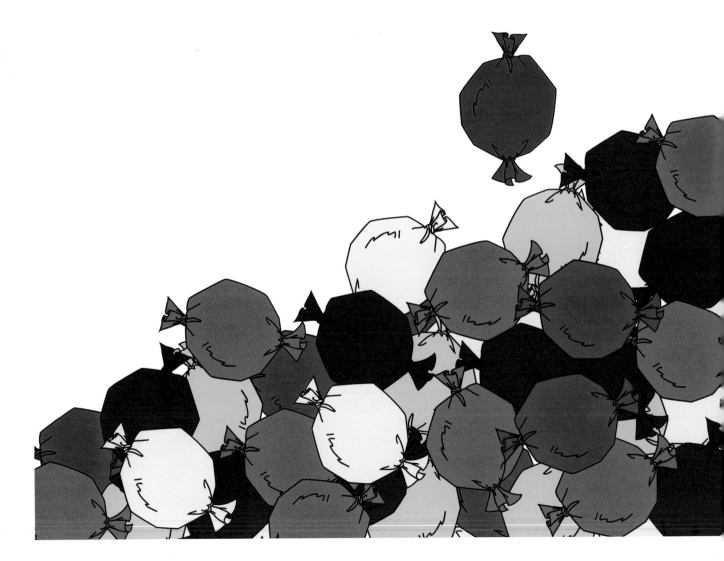

This book belongs to

_____

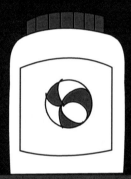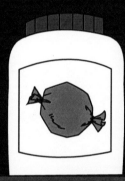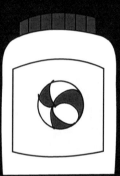

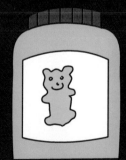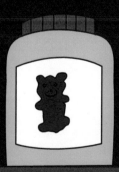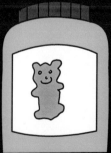

In Moderation

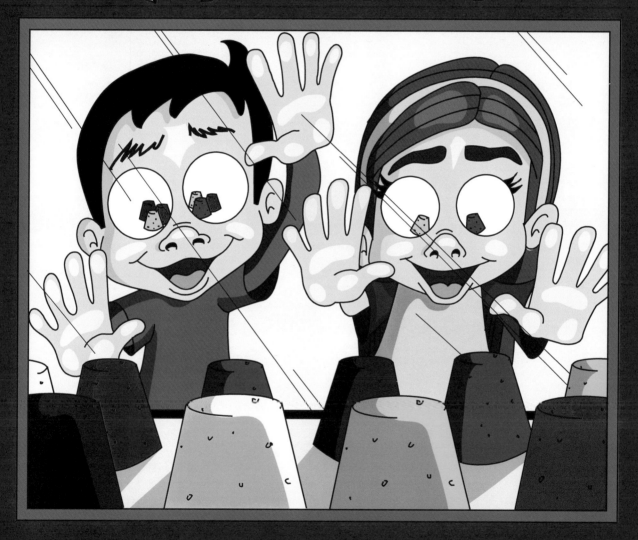

Written by: Antonio Braccioforte
Illustrated by: Matthew M. Keown

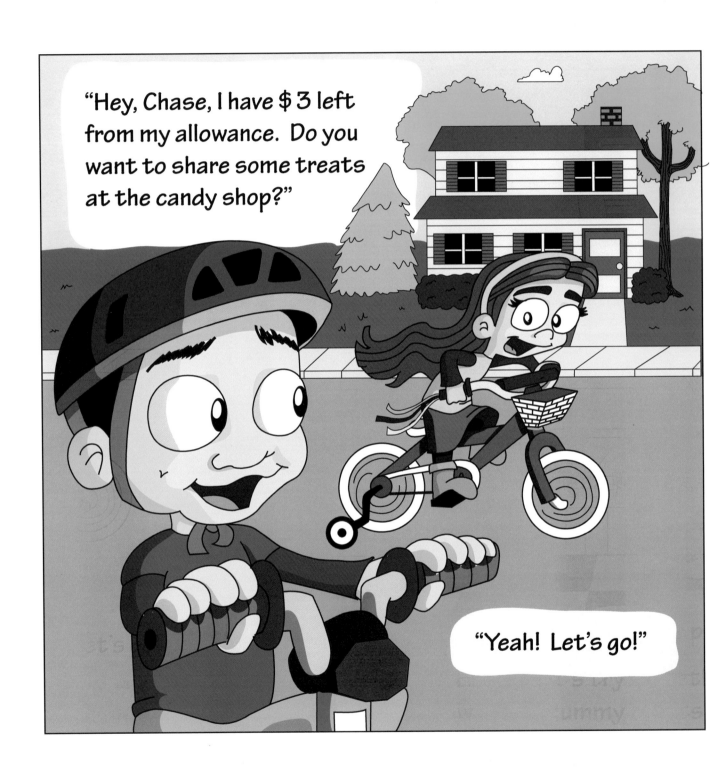

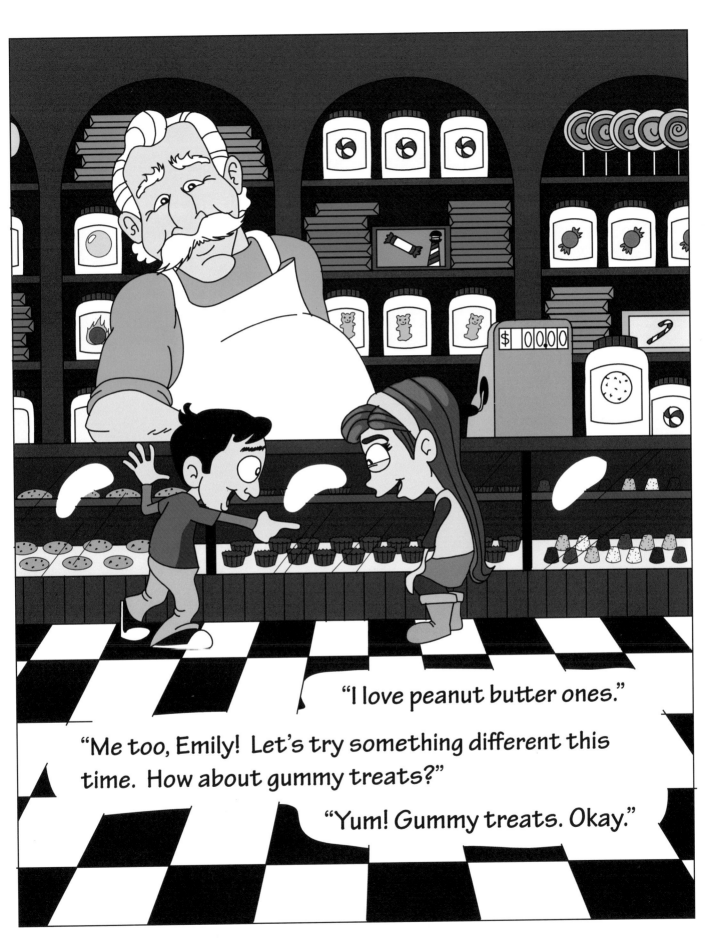

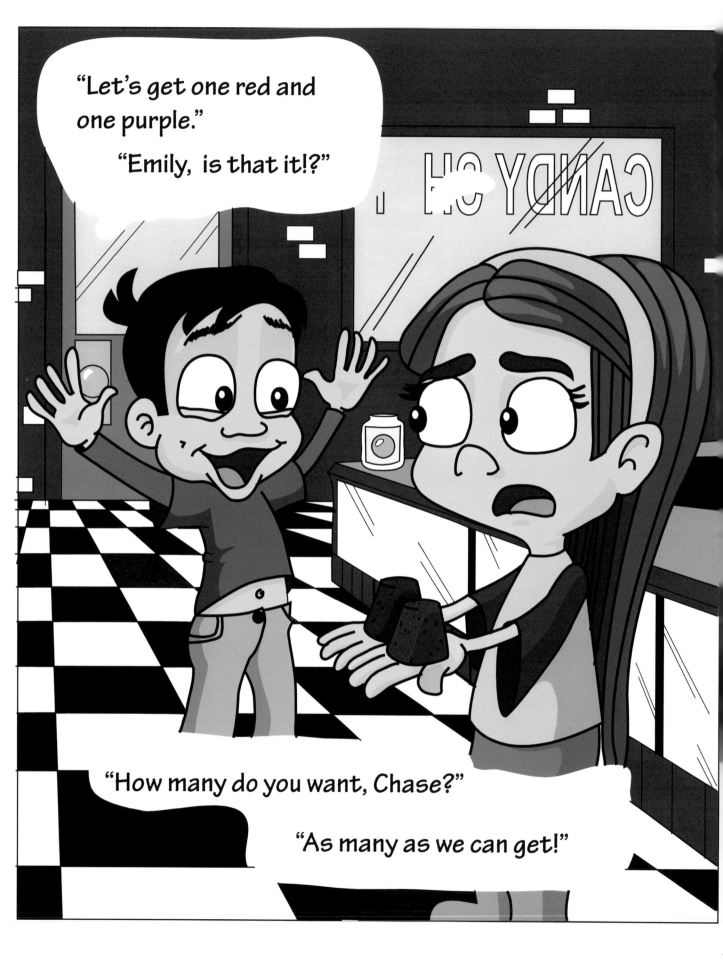

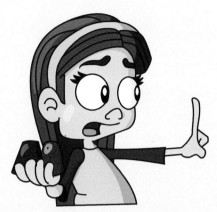
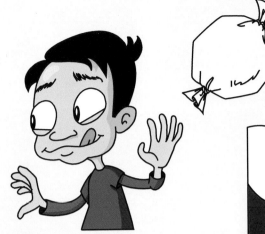

"If we eat too much, we'll get sick and our teeth will go bad!"

"But, Emily, it's candy! What do you mean?"

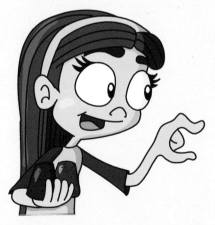
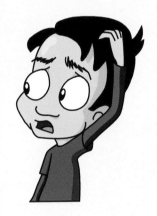

"Chase, my mom says it's okay to eat candy, but 'in moderation'."

"What does 'in moderation' mean?"

"In moderation means that we can eat candy, but we should NOT eat too much at one time."

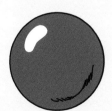
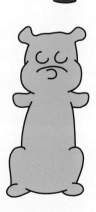

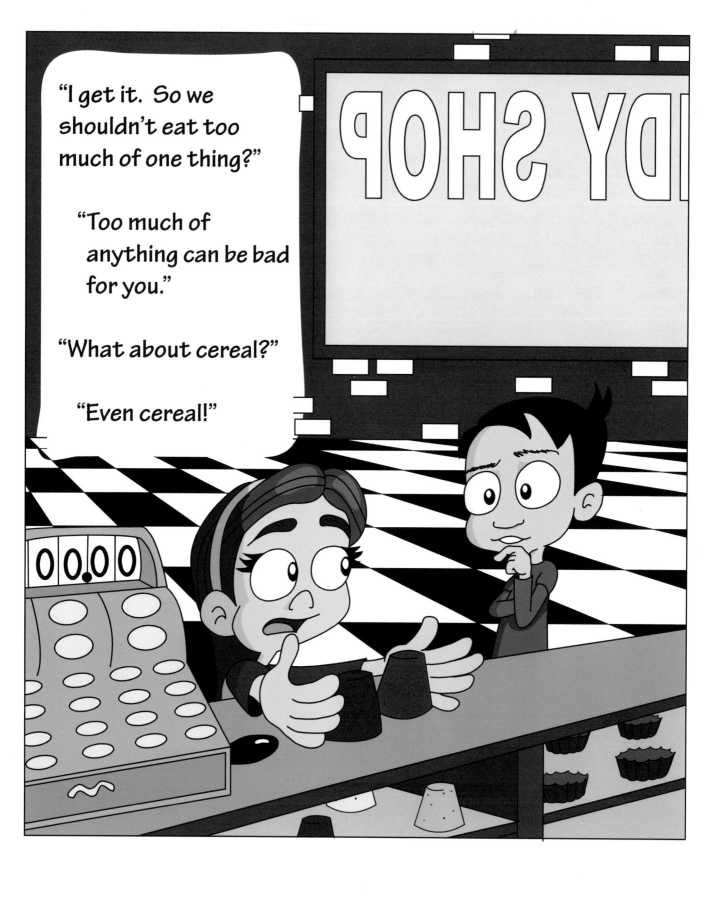

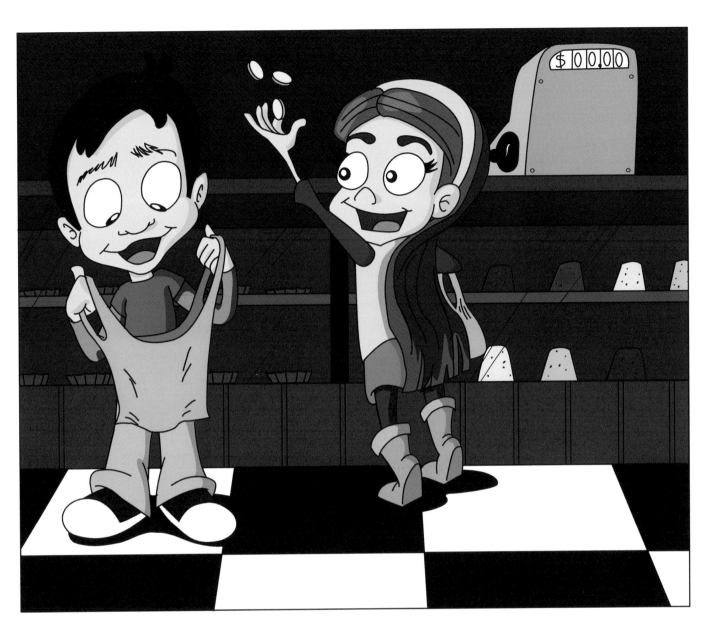

"You're right, Emily, let's get one for each of us."

"Okay, Chase. We can come back next time and get those peanut butter treats."

"Okay, but I'll save my allowance and buy them for us."

"Thanks, Chase. That sounds great!"

"And we'll only get one treat each, right, Emily?"

"Yep, that's what my mom says: 'In moderation'!"

"In moderation!"

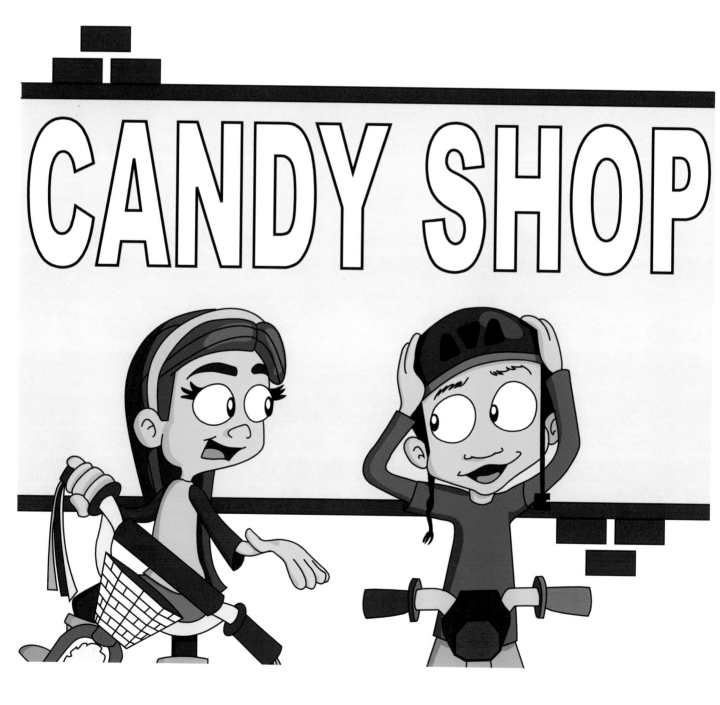

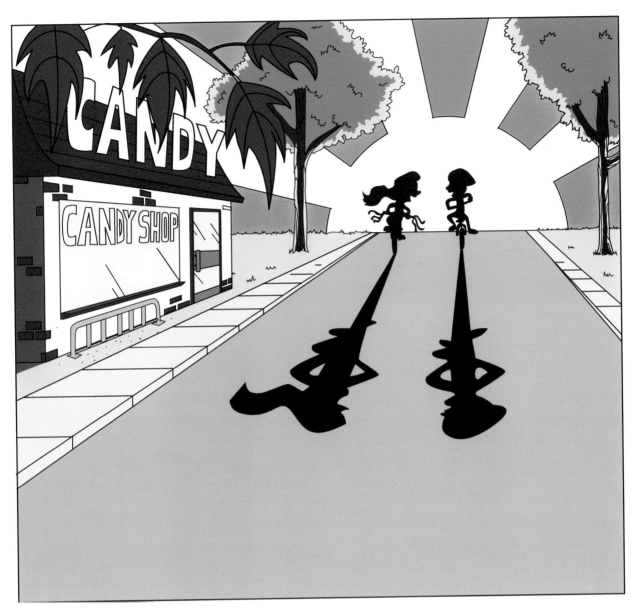

"You know, Chase, my mom tells me other good stuff too."

"Maybe I should listen to my mom more."

"Yeah, moms really do know a lot."

"One thing at a time, Emily...one thing at a time."

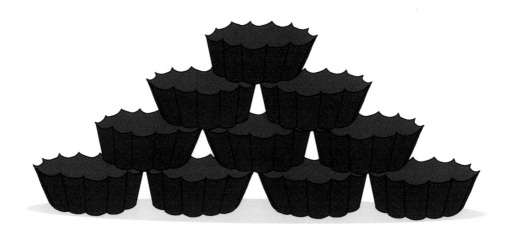

LaVergne, TN USA
31 October 2010
202864LV00003B